Bodybuilding

Meal Plans, Recipes And Bodybuilding Nutrition Know How To Eat For: Strength, Muscle And Fitness

2nd Edition

By

Nicholas Bjorn

Table of Contents

Introduction

Everyone dreams of having a perfectly shaped body. For a long time now, you may have wanted to get in shape, but you just do not have the time to do so. Every time you schedule a workout session at the gym, work or life gets in the way, which makes it increasingly difficult for you to achieve that fit physique.

Now is not the time to worry because there is a solution to make those muscles grow without relying on workout exercises alone. If you are too busy to visit the gym regularly but have been dreaming of achieving that perfectly shaped body, this book is for you.

I want to thank you and congratulate you for downloading the book, ***"Bodybuilding: Meal Plans, Recipes and Bodybuilding Nutrition: Know How to Eat For: Strength, Muscle and Fitness."***

This book contains proven steps and strategies on how to grow your muscles and have a fit figure without exerting too much effort on workout exercises. It provides you with a clear guide on the food that you must eat in order to achieve your dream body.

The first chapter of this book contains information on bodybuilding and its importance. The second chapter begins by informing you about the nutrients necessary to make your muscles grow, as well as provides examples of foods that contain these nutrients. The third chapter shares the characteristics of a good nutrition plan. Chapters four, five, and six contain good meal plans for breakfast, lunch, and dinner, respectively. Finally, chapter seven warns you about the food that you should avoid eating.

Thanks again for downloading this book, and I hope you enjoy it!

Chapter 1 – Bodybuilding and Its Importance

Bodybuilding is an activity that makes use of resistance exercises to develop and control your musculature. Bodybuilding has significant effects on many aspects of your life. It improves not only your physical health, but also your mental and emotional state. We have heard of a lot of people testifying that their whole lives have improved after focusing on bodybuilding. This chapter will share the importance of bodybuilding and reveal why it is beneficial to exert your time and effort on it.

Bodybuilding is important for the following reasons:

- *Bodybuilding makes you stronger*. Bodybuilding makes your muscles denser, and consequently, stronger. As a person engages himself or herself in bodybuilding, his or her muscles become bigger, thereby allowing him or her to lift heavier things. Of course, a person who engages in bodybuilding shines in activities that require strength. However, one should not put too much effort on making his or her muscles grow. As muscle mass increases, mobility and motion may be restricted.

- *Body fat is trimmed.* Given that bodybuilding requires workout exercises and weightlifting activities, fat is burned. In relation to this, a bodybuilding nutrition plan prevents you from eating food that has too much fat in it. This helps you maintain and develop a better physique and therefore allows you to achieve your bodybuilding goals.

- *Bodybuilding trains you to become disciplined.*

Bodybuilding is not an easy activity. You cannot just start whenever you want and then stop whenever you feel like doing so. If you truly want to achieve your bodybuilding goals, you must be passionate and disciplined. Your bodybuilding nutrition plan will restrict you from eating particular kinds of food, and you will be trained to follow this plan strictly. When you are required to work out at a specific time during the week, you will get used to doing so. Through bodybuilding, you will be able to discipline yourself and thus learns to manage your time.

- *Bodybuilding is a fulfilling activity*. There may be a lot of difficulties that you would face initially, but after you have devoted your time and effort to bodybuilding, you will be able to appreciate it. Bodybuilding produces results that will make you want to engage in it repeatedly. Through passion and proper discipline, you will benefit from the many physical, mental, and social effects that bodybuilding brings. It will not only make you stronger physically, but you will also feel a lot better about yourself. You will gain self-esteem and self-confidence. Although you may feel like giving up when you begin engaging yourself in bodybuilding activities, don't forget that choosing to continue is the only way to avoid regret.

Mentioned above are just some of the benefits that highlight the importance of bodybuilding. Without a doubt, bodybuilding is a worthwhile activity. It may be demanding, but it is only because it produces results that are truly fulfilling. Now that you know about the importance of bodybuilding, the next thing to do is to identify the kinds of nutrients that the body needs in order for your muscles to grow.

Chapter 2 – Nutrients Needed for Bodybuilding

The goals of bodybuilding can never be truly achieved through weightlifting exercises alone. Diet plays a significant role in realizing your bodybuilding goals. In bodybuilding, it is necessary that you accompany exercises with proper diet and nutrition. This chapter will inform you about the nutrients that your body needs for bodybuilding. At the same time, you will find examples of the kinds of food that contain these nutrients in order to guide you in making your nutrition plan.

In bodybuilding, it is necessary that your body gets the following nutrients:

Carbohydrates. Many people have a misconception that in order to burn fat, you must only consume minimal amounts of carbohydrates. This is not true. Carbohydrates are the primary energy source of our body. Science suggests that 50% of the food we eat should contain carbohydrates. They help a person cope with the rigors of hard training.

Protein. Protein is necessary for the growth and repair of tissues inside the body. It is a secondary source of energy that is burned and utilized when a person eats too little carbs. Proteins are composed of amino acids that are helpful in maintaining the body tissues.

Fat. Fats are the only source of fatty acids needed by the body. Without fatty acids, proper skin maintenance (particularly regeneration) would be impossible. The production of hormones would also be affected negatively. Fats are categorized into two, namely, saturated and unsaturated. They also serve as sources of energy to help you cope with the difficulty of doing exercise.

Vitamins. Vitamins are used as fuel and do not provide calories to the body. They serve as metabolic regulators and are responsible for the production of energy, growth, maintenance, and repair. There are a lot of identified vitamins, and they all have beneficial health effects on the body. Although intake of vitamins is healthy, excessive amounts can be detrimental to your health. Intake of vitamins should thus be moderated.

Minerals. These are inorganic compounds needed by the body in order to build teeth and bones, as well as to form hormones and other blood cells.

Now that you know the nutrients that your body needs for bodybuilding, you should be able to identify the kinds of food that contain these nutrients. The second part of this chapter gives you a list of foods rich in these nutrients.

Egg whites. Egg whites are the best-known source of protein. You will hardly find any bodybuilder who does not include egg whites in his or her diet. Egg whites also contain vitamins and minerals, as well as a few carbohydrates.

Fish. Bodybuilders often avoid fatty food, but fish, despite being fatty, is healthy. Fish also contains fatty acids, such as omega-3, that are actually helpful to the body. Fish is also a source of protein. These nutrients can usually be found in tuna, trout, salmon, and sardines.

Chicken and/or Turkey. Almost all bodybuilders have chicken and/or turkey in their nutrition plans. This is because chicken is a source of high-quality protein. It also has less trans-fat and saturated fats than other kinds of food.

Beans and Legumes. Beans and legumes are high-quality sources of fiber and protein. Fiber helps the body regulate its bowel movement, which is necessary to promote healthy bodybuilding activity. Some people immediately resort to lean meat, and it is often a neglected fact that beans and legumes are good sources of protein, too.

Water. While you are so concerned about the food that you need to eat, you may have forgotten that your body is composed of 70% water. Because you're sweating a lot every time you're working out, your body loses a great deal of water. Of course, it is necessary that you replace it by drinking plenty of water. This will help you stay hydrated.

Now that you know the kinds of food that you need to eat, it is time to prepare a nutrition plan. To come up with a good one, you must keep the things mentioned in the next chapter in mind.

Chapter 3 – Characteristics of a Good Nutrition Plan for Bodybuilding

Making a meal plan is not always easy. There are things to consider in order to achieve your bodybuilding goals fully. This chapter will teach you the characteristics of a good nutrition program for bodybuilding. Without further ado, here are the key qualities of a proper muscle-bulking meal plan:

1. It should focus on small meals and portions rather than large ones. Your metabolism increases when you eat small meals frequently rather than eat one large meal per day. Increased metabolism results in an increase in the capability to burn more fat. It is advisable that you eat four to six meals a day, with intervals of two to three hours.

2. Meals should contain protein, carbohydrates and fats. In order to achieve the desired results, you must observe a balanced diet with the correct ratio of these three nutrients. The correct ratio, as science suggests, is 40% protein, 40% carbohydrates, and 20% fats.

3. Your nutrition program should be compatible with the other aspects of your life. It must contain meal plans that suit your lifestyle and are applicable for a long period of time. Necessary changes should only be minimal. Moreover, it would be difficult for you to adapt to a new nutrition plan every couple of weeks. It is important that you are consistent so that you will achieve your desired goals.

4. Your meal plan should be designed in accordance with your bodybuilding goals. In other words, you must first specify your

bodybuilding goals before you begin creating a meal plan. How much muscle do you want to grow? Which part of your body would you like to become more muscular? This is important to note because there are meal plans especially designed to achieve particular results.

5. Meal ingredients should be accessible. There are meal plans with dishes that are too complicated that you would no longer know where to find the ingredients. Make sure that when you design your meal plan, the ingredients are simple yet healthy. Remember that your nutrition plan should be applicable for the rest of your life, which is why it is important that you have easy access to the ingredients.

Now that you know the characteristics of a good meal plan, the next step is to create your own. The succeeding chapters will share sample meal plans that you could use for five days.

Chapter 4 – Shopping List

Normally whenever anyone mentions bodybuilding people tend to think of heavy weight training and other related things. Beginners and amateur enthusiasts thus often frequent their local gyms and train like lunatics. This training is worthless if you do not pair it with a proper and well-researched diet plan. Your 'I am eating healthier than before' excuse will not work if you are trying to build muscle. It is also possible that you will lose weight and gain muscle without following a proper diet but these results will stop at some point..

To build muscle you need to follow a specific diet and nutrients in specific amounts as well. The basics of diet and nutrition are covered in the subsequent chapters but before that, in this chapter, we will have a look at the things that you need to buy before starting a muscle building diet.

Most of the things mentioned in this list are easily available in any grocery store or supermarket. You can stock most of these things but do not store perishable goods for long time. If possible, follow the list to the T, unless of course you are allergic to something. In such a case consult a good dietician and ask what you can replace that item with.

Here is an exhaustive list of things that you should buy and things that you should not buy. Ideally, you should follow your diet plan to the T, but a cheat meal twice a month will not cause much harm. For the ease of reference the list has been divided into sections according to nutrients, so if you feel that you are lacking protein you can make up for that protein by referring to the protein section and buy things that are rich in protein.

Protein

What to Buy:

- Eggs: Eggs are the best source of protein. All kinds of eggs are okay to eat. Normally egg whites should be preferred but yolks are fine too.

- Chicken Breasts or Cutlets (Skinless): Chicken, like eggs, is a rich source of protein. Buy good quality, inexpensive and lean chicken. You can cook this in a variety of ways. As chicken is perishable always buy it fresh and use it immediately.

- Ground Turkey (Lean): Although ground turkey is a bit more expensive it is as a good change when you get bored of eating chicken; you can rely on Turkey as a rich source or protein. Once again, you should always buy fresh turkey and use it immediately.

- Steak: Avoid steak if you are on a very strict diet. If not, then you should not miss steak as it is a good source of protein and fat. Only buy fresh and lean steak.

- Mignon Filet: Very expensive but tasty as well. Buy it occasionally to treat your palate.

- Buffalo: This is definitely the most expensive meat on this list. Only buy fresh and lean buffalo meat.

- Flounder: Flounder is an inexpensive breed of fish that also happens to be very tasty. Buy it fresh as opposed to the frozen variety, but when you have no option, you can go for the frozen ones.

- Cod: Another inexpensive breed of fish that is packed with proteins and is tasty as well.

- Pollock: A lean fish. Is found easily in the seafood section of the supermarket.
- Salmon: Salmon is famous for its protein richness and taste. It is also rather fatty so eat it in moderation. Wild salmon is more expensive than bred salmon.
- Tuna (canned): Canned tuna is once again a tasty, inexpensive, and lean fish. However if you are on a low sodium diet you should avoid this fish or eat it in moderation. In addition, only buy fish that is canned in water and not in oil.
- Turkey Bacon: Bacon is generally not allowed on a bodybuilding diet so as a replacement you should consider buying turkey bacon. Eat it sparingly- twice a month is more than enough as a treat for your taste buds.
- Ground Beef (Lean): Buy good quality, 90% lean beef. It is a high source of protein and can be consumed in off-season.
- Paneer: Paneer is a form of cottage cheese that is popular in the Indian Subcontinent. It is slow digesting so you can feel full and satiated for a long time. It is versatile and you can make a variety of things with it.
- Pork Tenderloin: Buy good quality, low cost, lean tenderloins, as they are a great source of proteins.
- Bass (Sea): Expensive but tasty. You can eat it occasionally.
- Swordfish: Expensive but tasty. You can eat it occasionally.

What Not to Buy:

- Skinned Chicken: Only buy skinless chicken, as the chicken skin is full of unhealthy fats that are best avoided.
- Breaded Chicken: The breadcrumbs add unnecessary carbs to your diet.
- Deli Meat: Is full of additives and preservatives and is generally of low quality.
- Bacon: As said earlier avoid bacon. It is tasty but very fatty and thus can wreck havoc on your diet plan. Not a good friend for heart related issues
- Ground Beef (Fatty): Lean ground beef should be preferred over fatty one because as the name suggests regular beef contains high amounts of fats.
- Fatty Cuts of Meat: Go for lean cuts of meats always. Regular cuts generally contain unnecessary fats that are not good for your diet.

Carbohydrates

What to Buy:

- Steel Cut Oats: Steel Cut Oats are a high source of carbs that are fulfilling and will keep you satiated for a long time. Ideal for breakfast.
- Oatmeal: Very healthy like oats. It is a slow digesting food thus it will keep you satiated for a long time. Ideal food for breakfast.

- Fruits: All fresh fruits are healthy sources of carbs but some contain more carbs as compared to others. Blueberries are a rich source of antioxidants. Bananas contain high amount of carbs that are good for energy especially after heavy workouts. Bananas contain simple carbs so they are easy digesting fruits.

- Vegetables: Like fruits all vegetables are okay to eat. You cannot go wrong with vegetables. Although all have various health benefits, green and leafy vegetables should be your priority while dieting. These vegetables are high in iron, low in calories, fiber rich and tasty as well. Eat green vegetables in every meal. Sweet potatoes are a good source of fiber and carbs and are healthier as compared to regular potatoes. Eat them boiled with a little splenda. Yams can be eaten instead.

- Brown Rice: Although some people do not really bother to eat rice but if you are a rice eating person you should always opt for brown rice to white rice. Brown rice contains slow digesting carbs and thus keeps you satiated for long.

- Bread (Whole wheat bread): Although you should avoid bread altogether, but if you love bread you should eat the whole-wheat variety as compared to the other varieties. Read labels carefully before buying bread.

- Cream of Rice and Cream of Wheat: both of these things can be used instead of normal white rice. These carbs digest fast as compared to the ones mentioned above.

What not to Buy:

- Cereal: Gone are the days when cereals where considered a healthy breakfast, now most of the companies add high amounts of chemicals and sugar. Instead of eating cereal, eat oatmeal. You can enhance the taste of oatmeal by adding various fruits such as berries, apples, bananas etc to it.

- Candy/Toffee: This is obvious. Candy is loaded with harmful sugar that can wreck havoc on your diet and health. Avoid it.

- Crisps: Crisps, chips and French fries are loaded with unnecessary fats and simple carbs. They are harmful to your health and diet. Avoid them.

- Ice Cream and Fatty Milkshakes: Both of these things are loaded with harmful sugar so you should avoid them. Opt for smoothies instead.

- Soda: Any kind of soda is harmful for your diet routine. Steer clear from regular soda, low sugar soda, diet soda etc.

- Juice: Fruit juice may help you in other forms of diet but ideally, you should avoid them in this diet. Eat the whole fruit instead.

Fats

What to Buy:

- Olive Oil/ Flaxseed Oil: Olive oil is one of the best fats that you can add to your diet. Buy regular, virgin, and extra virgin olive oil and use them accordingly. If you want to go for an inexpensive alternative go for flaxseed oil.

- Almond Butter: This butter derived from almonds is healthier than the regular butter.
- Fish oil: Fish oil is nutrient rich and has a peculiar taste as well.
- Pecans: Rich source of good fats.
- Almonds: Rich source of good fats.
- Cashews: Rich source of good fats.
- Walnuts: Rich source of good fats.
- Unsalted Pistachio: Rich source of good fats.
- Unsalted Peanuts: Rich source of good fats.
- Avocados: Rich source of good fats.

Peanut Butter: Only buy natural and unprocessed butter. You can add this to protein shakes. It is a rich source of protein and fats.

Chapter 5 – Do's And Don'ts

This chapter contains some important Do's and Don'ts of bodybuilding and nutrition in general. Most of these things are easy to follow and thus can be followed by almost everyone. The mistakes in the Don'ts section are rookie mistakes yet many people frequently repeat them. Avoid them and stay on your regime for a healthy and active body.

Now let us have a look at the Do's and Don'ts of bodybuilding.

DO's

- Prepare in Advance:

  Instead of making your meals in hurry, prepare for them in advance and if possible cook it in advance as well. Cooking a meal in advance or being well prepared will help you to avoid fast food and untimely healthy snacking. Make a weekly plan and follow it to the T. You can also cook in advance on Mondays, Wednesdays and Sundays and can eat the leftovers on the other days (do not make anything perishable). Keep oatmeal, eggs etc ready for your morning breakfast the night before so you don't skip breakfast due to lack of cooking time. Remember, your breakfast is the most important meal of the day. You don't want to eat readymade cereal for something that is the MOST important meal. Eggs, oats, brown bread, fruits and smoothies etc. are ideal breakfast to kick start your day.

- Divide Portions

  Divide your portions according to the size. Pack these in appropriate containers. If you are not sure of sizes, you can follow this chart:

	Portion	What does it look like?
1.	Meat- 1 oz	A regular matchbox
2.	Fish-4 oz	A regular Checkbook
3.	Cheese- 1 1/2 oz	A large dice
4.	Potato - medium	A computer mouse
5.	Peanut Butter - 2 tbsp	A ping pong ball
6.	Pasta- 1 cup	A tennis Ball
7.	Bagel	A hockey puck
8.	Meat 4 oz	A bar of soap
9.	Meat 9 oz	A thin notebook

Prepare these and put them in appropriately sized containers. Put these in the freezer for future use. Ideally, you should feel hungry after 3 hours of your last meals; if you do not then you have consumed extra calories.

- Keep Water Ready

  We all know that water forms a major component of human body. 74% of your brain is water, 75% of muscles are water, and 83 % of blood is water as well.

  Drinking healthy amount of water is essential for good

health. Your body needs water for digestion, blood circulation and almost every important bodily process. It also serves as a detoxifier and keeps your organs healthy. Try to drink at least a gallon of water every day. Carrying a bottle always in your bag at all times will help you to consume water.

- Be consistent

Consistency is an important factor not only in bodybuilding but also in almost every activity that you do. You should be consistent with your diet plan and your exercise routine. Following a simple diet plan regularly is much better than following a well-planned diet occasionally. The first one will show better results than the latter.

Being consistent with your diet plan is also good for your self-esteem. You will feel good about yourself and your level of dedication will increase too. You will develop a positive outlook towards life.

Remember each hit counts when you are trying to chop down a tree.

DON'Ts

- Making Excuses

Sometimes you simply cannot resist eating and give in to your cravings. This is okay but what most people do after this is not. People start making excuses for this failure and most of the times these excuses are pathetic.

“I was feeling sick so I eat my favorite food”

"Donuts comfort me"

"I was feeling sad so I ate this"

All of these excuses are extremely lame and biased. Not only these excuses give you a reason to start eating unhealthy food again they also give you a false sense of security. These excuses will mess up your results and in turn you will blame the diet and your exercise regime.

Remember only a bad worker fights with his tools.

- Comparison and Competition:

  Healthy competition is generally a good thing in any aspect, as it keeps you motivated and active. In bodybuilding, there will always be people who will be stronger, bigger, leaner, and more muscular than you. You need to accept this because not all bodies are same. Everyone is different. If you keep on comparing yourself with others, you will never achieve your goals. Not only is this unnecessary but also stupid as it can harm you.

  Instead of competing with others, compete with yourself. Try to beat your personal best in every field. Measure your progress and keep a track of it. Do not hesitate to make changes in your plans.

  Do not copy other people's regime and diet plans. Most of the diet plans are specially prepared for the individual. These plans will not help you. Devise your own plan. Bodybuilding is an art where your body is your medium. Only you know your limits and your perquisites; use them accordingly.

- Not Tracking Your Progress

  One of the rookie mistakes than beginners always seem to do is not keeping an eye on their progress. Bodybuilding and dieting is a matter of rhythm and planning, you need to follow it perfectly. Keeping a track of your progress helps to follow your plans effectively. Bodybuilding is not a mindless job you need to be dedicated to see results.

  Always maintain a journal and track your exercise regime as well as your diet plan. Measure everything and track everything. This will help you to adjust your diet and exercise routine. Having a tracked plan is like the base of a building. If your base is good your building will stand erect else it will crumble to pieces.

- Unrealistic Expectations

  If you think that you can get a ripped and Greek God like body by following a fad diet or taking some kind of supplements then you are in for a rude surprise. Not only these diets don't work but they also cause much harm to your body. You cannot expect to start lifting 300 pounds weights in your first week of weight training by gulping down a protein shake with supplements. Similarly, you cannot lose 50 lbs. in 3 weeks by dieting. All of these are simply myths that you should steer away from.

  Only patience, dedication, and consistency can help you to achieve your goals. Changing the shape and size of your body is not a simple job. You cannot achieve your dream body in a week. Incidentally, your dream body might be just a dream. Most of us dream of unrealistic bodies that are just impossible to achieve.

- Too Much

  Too much is too bad. Too much of everything including dieting and training/exercise is a harmful thing, it can wreak havoc on your body.

  Beginners often think that extra exercise and a strict diet plan will help them see instant results. This practice often shows zero results and is harmful as well.

  Bodybuilding is all about exercise, diet, and rest. The third part of the trio is as much important as the former two. You need to give your body ample rest after training and dieting. Your body needs recovery time, if you do not provide it with this you start overtraining which can induce fatigue, muscle pain, lack of motivation, exhaustion, injuries, insomnia etc.

- Too Little

  Like too much, too less is too bad too.

  People who have over-trained in the past are the ones who commit this mistake quite often. As said in the previous point, rest is very important as it gives your body time to restore and rejuvenate. Some people overdo this; they rest too much, and train too less. This results into no results.

  You cannot achieve a good body by resting 20 days a month, and training and dieting for the remaining 10 days. You will just fool yourself and will blame the regime.

- Supplements

  Open any general health magazine and you will find that it is full of advertisements for supplements of all kinds. This has led to the popularity of supplements and nowadays even trained professionals have started using them. So, do you really need to take supplements to get a chiseled body?

The answer is no of course. You can develop a chiseled, healthy, and perfect physique by following a healthy nutritional plan and exercise regime. Some people even manage to do this by following a strict vegan diet!

So, are supplements worthless? No, supplements are not worthless; they can help you achieve your goals, but more than often you can easily achieve them without any help of any supplements.

Nothing is instant in this world. You need to work hard to get that perfect body.

No Plan

Diet is the most critical part of your bodybuilding routine. You can do all kinds of workout but they will not show any results if you do not pair them with a good nutritional plan. Your body is a machine and you need to fuel it properly and regularly.

Most people love to exercise. This is commonly seen in the 'gym freaks'. People consider exercise fashionable, enjoyable, and fun. However, more than often these people do not see results. This is because they do not accompany their exercise routine with a good and well-made diet plan.

It is not that people do not know the benefits of a good and well-planned diet and nearly everyone knows the six meals diet. Majority of people do not healthy because of time. People generally complain that they do not get enough time to eat properly and thus eat fast food. This is just a myth.

Fast food is just a myth; it takes equal amount of time to eat a regular diet and a fast food diet. Yes, cooking a regular meal does take more time but compare it with the disadvantages of fast food, and you will get my point that fast food is basically nothing but a short cut to an unhealthy life.

Whenever you are free, cook some healthy meals in advance and pack it up. This will help you to plan your meals effectively and you will not be tempted to eat fast food. This will reduce the time you spend in the kitchen and will thus help you to achieve your weight loss goals with ease.

Chapter 6 – Simple Tips To Follow

In this chapter, you will find tips related to nutrition and overall bodybuilding routine. These tips are well tested. Following these tips will help your bodybuilding routine and can help you to avoid rookie mistakes. Now let us look at these tips one at a time.

- Always consult a physician or dietician before starting any diet routine. Your dietician should approve your diet plan. Do not follow any fad diet.

- As soon as you start dieting, start monitoring your vital statistics. Keep a constant record of these.

- Remember, no two people are alike; everyone is different. A specific person can lose a lot of weight by following some form of diet but you probably will not. This is perfectly normal. This is why you should consult a good dietician and get a custom-made plan for yourself.

- If you have some kind of heart condition or related disorders you should consult with your specialist before starting any kind of diet or exercise routine.

- You may see certain side effects such as muscle pain, cravings etc in the beginning but do not worry, as these are normal. Nevertheless, if these symptoms persist, stop your routine and consult a doctor as soon as possible.

- To curb your cravings for sweets, eat fruits regularly. Fruits are full of nutrients and good sugar. Keep a stash of fruits in your house.

- Take your time to eat i.e. eat slowly. Slow eating fools

your body into believing that it is full. Enjoy your meals and eat it at a dinner table instead of sitting in front of the television. Do not eat until you feel full or bloated; your brain gets signal that you are full a bit late and by then usually you end up overeating.

- Increase the intake of insoluble fiber. Fiber not only helps you to feel full fast but it is also good for digestion. Many times digestion suffers when you start a new diet. Consuming a healthy amount of fiber will help you to regulate your digestive system.

- Increase your intake of water. Replace all of your beverages with water. If you do not like to drink plain water, infuse it with fruits for taste and a dash of nutrition.

- Have an occasional treat to keep your cravings at bay. However, do not over indulge.

- Look for healthy and tasty recipes online according to the availability of fresh ingredients. These recipes will help you to curb your cravings.

- Never ever, skip breakfast. Breakfast is called breakfast because you literally break your night long fast. It thus is the most important meal of your day. A rich breakfast will keep you active throughout the day and will satiate your cravings as well.

- Exchange ice creams for mashed frozen bananas. Instead of using spaghetti use juliennes of zucchini, carrots etc. instead of using mayonnaise use hummus, seasoned tomato puree etc. Instead of fried potato chips use baked carrot chips. Use silken tofu instead of cream. Use almond milk instead of simple milk. Use brown bread instead of white bread.

- Use small plates instead of large ones, so you don't pile food up as a force of habit.
- Chew gum whenever you feel sudden craving for something sweet. Only use sugar free gum.
- Do not add too much salt to your meals.
- Plan a goal and follow it.
- To motivate yourself try reading motivational books, listening your favorite songs etc. These actions may seem small but they help you take your mind off of the food craving and help you with your weight loss goals
- Get a sipper and fill it with water. Sip water throughout the day to keep yourself hydrated.
- Use tools and Smartphone apps to gauge your progress.
- Celebrate each little achievement with simple (low fat) treats.
- Avoid excuses.
- Generally avoid visiting restaurants. If you have to visit a restaurant then follow these steps. Check the website of the restaurant beforehand. These websites generally have nutritional information about their menu. Choose the items that not affect your diet drastically and order them when you go to the restaurant. If your restaurant does not have a website then order only broiled, boiled, baked, grilled or steamed dishes. Avoid anything deep-fried. Eat a small salad or something healthy at home before going to the restaurant to avoid overeating. Ask for sauces on

the side. Instead of skipping your dessert altogether or eating it alone, try sharing it with others.

- Avoid stress. Stress is not only bad for health but it also induces binge eating or eating for pleasure. Try some stress busting exercises or activities to keep you active.
- Sleep for 6-8 hours daily. As said earlier rest and recovery time is an essential part of any healthy weight-loss system. Sleep is the best rest you can get. Sleep early and wake up early as well. Early morning air is good for your health.
- Do not eat unplanned meals. Unplanned meals result into overeating that in turn ruins your diet.
- Set reminders on your phone to drink water. You can also download some free apps that remind you to drink water.
- Maintain a positive mindset about your food. Do not consider cooking as a task but think of it as a pleasurable activity. Relish your food.
- Recharge your body after each workout session. A good protein shake or protein rich snack will prevent fatigue. Do not choose unhealthy and fried snacks.

If possible, get a dieting partner.

Chapter 7 – Meal Plan: Breakfast

This chapter features a sample seven-day breakfast meal plan. Mentioned in this chapter are the kinds of food that you may include in your breakfast for each day of the week. This chapter also contains sample meals and recipes that you can prepare at home.

Day 1:

- 1 banana
- ½ cup of oat bran
- 1 egg yolk
- 6 hardboiled egg whites

Day 2:

- 1 cup of cottage cheese
- 1 cup of yogurt
- 1 tablespoon of flaxseed
- 1 bunch of red grapes

Day 3:

- 1 cup of oats
- 1 apple
- ½ ounce of walnuts

- 1 cup of cottage cheese

Day 4:

- ½ cup of rolled oats
- 1 cup of blueberries
- 1 cup of cottage cheese
- Cinnamon
- 1 tablespoon of flaxseed

Day 5:

- 9 egg whites
- 1 cup of spinach leaves
- 2 strips of turkey bacon
- 1 apple
- 1 garlic
- 1 grapefruit

Day 6:

- 1 English muffin
- 6 egg whites
- 1 egg yolk
- 1 grapefruit

- 2 strips of turkey bacon

Day 7:

- ½ cup of oat bran
- ½ ounce of walnuts
- 1 cup of frozen berries
- 1 scoop of protein
- ½ tablespoon of flaxseed

Sample Breakfast Recipes

Healthy Homemade Banana Split

This might sound new to you, but yes, a banana split happens to be a good and healthy breakfast for bodybuilders. It is a good source of protein and can thus help you boost your energy as you proceed with your cardiovascular routine. You will only need roughly seven ingredients, namely:

- 1 medium-sized banana
- 1 chopped strawberry
- ¾ cup Greek yogurt that is non-fat
- ½ scoop Dymatize ISO Protein
- 1 tablespoon of dark chocolate chips
- 1 large tablespoon of granola

To make your healthy homemade banana split:

1. Divide the medium-sized banana into two by slicing it in half lengthwise.
2. Put them on a clean plate or bowl.
3. Mix the ¾ cup non-fat Greek yogurt with the Dymatize ISO Protein and put them on top of the sliced banana.

The chopped strawberry, dark chocolate chips, and granola will serve as topping. This is a delicious breakfast that will not only satisfy your cravings, but will also help you realize your bodybuilding goals.

Healthy French Toast with Apples

French Toasts is a favorite of many people, particularly bodybuilders. This is a meal that you cannot afford to miss. If you are planning to spend your day doing leg workouts and other cardiovascular exercises, this is the perfect meal for you. There are only six ingredients needed, namely:

- 2 to 3 slices of grain or wheat bread
- 1 scoop of vanilla protein
- ¼ cup of almond milk
- 1 egg
- 1 egg white
- Cinnamon

To make it more delicious and healthy, you may opt to add slices of apples. This can easily be done because most of the ingredients are readily available at home. After you have gathered all the ingredients:

1. Have your bowl ready and mix in the egg, vanilla protein, almond milk, and cinnamon.
2. Soak the slices of bread one by one into the mixture.
3. Prepare your frying pan, and put a small amount of olive or coconut oil.
4. Cook each slice of wheat or grain bread until slightly browned.
5. Top the bread with sliced apples, and pour honey onto them if you want

Chapter 8 – Meal Plan: Lunch

This chapter shares a sample seven-day lunch meal plan. Mentioned in this chapter are the kinds of food that you may include in your lunch for every day of the week. Moreover, you can find sample meals and recipes that you can prepare at home.

Day 1:

- 1 cup of frozen blueberries
- 2 strips of turkey bacon
- 1 tablespoon of flaxseed
- 1 scoop of protein
- ½ cup of walnuts

Day 2:

- 2 strips of turkey bacon
- 3 ounces of grilled chicken
- ½ cup of mushrooms
- Balsamic vinegar
- 1 cup of chopped carrots

Day 3:

- 4 ounces of grilled chicken

- 3 cups of spinach leaves
- ½ cup of black beans
- 2 strips of turkey bacon
- Balsamic vinegar
- ½ cup of mushrooms

Day 4:

- 1 can of tuna
- 1 tablespoon of balsamic vinegar
- 1 piece of banana
- ½ cup of black beans

Day 5:

- 3 ounces of grilled chicken
- 1 whole-wheat tortilla
- ½ cup of shredded carrots
- 1 handful of spinach leaves
- ½ cup of hummus

Day 6:

- 3 cups of spinach leaves
- 4 ounces of grilled chicken

- Balsamic vinegar
- 1 cup of chopped carrots
- ½ cup of mushrooms

Day 7:

- 4 ounces of grilled chicken
- 2 slices of whole wheat bread
- 1 piece of orange
- 1 ounce of almonds
- Mustard
- Sliced lettuce

Sample Lunch Recipes

Cajun Tuna with Black Beans

Preparing this meal will only take you 15 to 20 minutes. It is simple and quick, yet healthy and effective. There are around eight ingredients needed to prepare this meal. They are as follows:

- Dark red or purple tuna
- A cup of cooked sushi rice
- A can of black beans
- Olive oil
- Chopped tomato
- Chopped ¼ onion
- Fresh cilantro

You will only need two cooking materials, namely, a small saucepan and a small skillet. To prepare this dish, follow these steps:

1. Prepare the rice.
2. Put the beans on the saucepan, and wait until they're warm.
3. Sprinkle Cajun seasoning onto the tuna until you get the flavor that you desire.
4. Put a small amount of oil onto the skillet, and cook both sides of the tuna.

5. Make sure that you do not overcook the fish because it will not be as tender as it needs to be if you cook it for more than two to three minutes per side.

6. If the rice has gotten cold, heat it in the microwave.

7. After the tuna is cooked, place it on a plate.

8. Sprinkle the beans, along with onions, cilantro, and chopped tomato, on top of the fish. After only 15 to 20 minutes of preparation and cooking time, your meal is now ready to be enjoyed.

Grilled Vegetables

This is a healthy, vegetarian meal for lunch. This meal can be prepared and cooked for about 25 to 30 minutes. These are the main ingredients that you will need to have:

- 1 eggplant
- 1 yellow squash
- 1 green zucchini
- 1 red bell pepper
- 1 peeled red onion
- 10 large mushrooms
- 1 bunch of asparagus
- ½ teaspoon of sea salt
- ¼ cup of olive oil
- 1 tablespoon of minced fresh garlic
- A pinch or two of pepper

For the cooking materials, you only need a small mixing bowl, a veggie grill basket, and two gallon-sized plastic bags. The steps that you need to do are:

1. Heat up the grill.
2. While the grill is heating, wash the vegetables and cut them in half or in small pieces.
3. Slice the onions, garlic, and other ingredients and keep their sizes consistent and make them look presentable.

4. Mix the pepper, salt, oil, and garlic, and put them in plastic bags. After the ingredients have been thoroughly mixed, put in the vegetables, and toss them together with the seasoning.

5. After they are completely and evenly mixed, put them in the basket and onto the grill.

6. Toss them once in a while for about ten minutes until they are perfectly cooked. Make sure that you do not overcook them in order to preserve the crispness.

7. To add to the taste, you may opt to sprinkle the vegetables with Parmesan cheese.

Chapter 9 – Meal Plan: Dinner

It's time for you to learn about dinner, particularly the muscle-boosting kind. By reading this chapter, you'll discover a sample dinner meal plan and several easy-to-prepare recipes.

Day 1:

- 3 ounces of grilled salmon
- 2 cups of steamed Swiss chard
- ¼ cup of brown rice

Day 2:

- 3 ounces of pork chop
- 1 cup of broccoli
- 1 medium-sized sweet potato
- 1 orange

Day 3:

- 4 ounces of turkey burger
- 1 cup of carrot sticks
- 1 cup of non-fat milk
- ½ cup of cooked quinoa

Day 4:

- 5 ounces of lean red meat
- 1 cup of cooked barley
- 1 whole chopped bell peppers
- ½ cup of spaghetti sauce
- ½ cup of mushrooms

Day 5:

- 3 ounces of pork chop
- 1 cup of asparagus
- 1 piece of sweet potato
- 1 cup of non-fat milk

Day 6:

- 4 ounces of grilled chicken
- 1 whole wheat tortilla
- 2 tablespoon of guacamole
- 1 cup of chopped bell peppers

Day 7:

- 1 slice of Canadian bacon
- 6 egg whites

- 1 pear
- 1 apple
- 1 ounce of cheese

Sample Dinner Recipes

Chicken and Vegetable Burritos

In only fifteen minutes, you can have a healthy and delicious meal prepared for dinner. To prepare chicken and vegetable burritos, you would need around nine simple ingredients. They are as follows:

- Boneless and skinless chicken breasts
- Cooked brown rice (optional)
- 1/3 cup of mushrooms
- ¼ red onion
- 1 tablespoon of olive oil
- ½ roasted bell pepper
- Low-carbohydrate tortillas
- Minced garlic

Prepare a medium-sized skillet and a microwave for cooking. Here are the steps in making chicken and vegetable burritos:

1. Cut the mushroom, pepper, garlic, and onion into thin slices.
2. After heating the oil, place these ingredients on the skillet. After cooking for around five minutes, add the sliced chicken.
3. Heat the tortillas in a microwave.
4. After everything has been cooked, roll the tortillas with the chicken in the middle (burrito-style). Enjoy a healthy and light dinner.

Lasagna

This is perhaps the quickest way of preparing healthy lasagna because it only takes 20 to 25 minutes. To prepare this lasagna, here are the ingredients that you will need:

- 1 pack of bowtie pasta
- 1 tablespoon of olive oil
- 1 teaspoon of minced fresh garlic
- ¼ cup of chopped onion
- 1 pound of lean ground beef
- Salt
- Pepper
- 1 cup of low-fat cheese
- 2 tablespoon of parmesan cheese

You will also need a large pasta pot and a skillet. To start off:

1. Boil water in the large pasta pot. After the water reaches a rapid boil, put in the bowtie pasta. Drain well.
2. For about five minutes, heat the oil, and then place the garlic and onion on the skillet. Add the beef, and cook everything well for ten minutes. Add salt and pepper to taste.
3. After doing this, add the cottage cheese. Mix the ingredients together until you achieve a sauce-like consistency.
4. When done, pour the sauce over the pasta, and mix well and evenly.

5. To make it taste even more delicious, sprinkle Parmesan cheese; your quick lasagna is ready.

Chapter 10 – Meal Plan: Snacks

In this chapter, you'll discover a seven-day snack meal plan that will definitely contribute to achieving your bodybuilding goals. Similar to previous chapters, you will also find some recipes, and you will learn about the kinds of food that you could eat for snacks.

Day 1:

- 1 cup of yogurt
- 1 bunch of red grapes
- 1 cup of cottage cheese
- 1 tablespoon of flaxseed

Day 2:

- 1 tablespoon of flaxseed
- 1 cup of blackberries
- Meal replacement shake

Day 3:

- 1 scoop of protein
- 1 banana
- 2 slices of whole wheat bread
- 1 tablespoon of peanut butter

Day 4:

- 1 garlic
- 6 egg whites
- 2 egg yolk
- 1 cup of chopped squash
- 3 cups of spinach leaves
- 1 whole grapefruit

Day 5:

- 1 cup of tea
- 1 cup of cottage cheese
- 1 cup of yogurt
- 1 tablespoon of flaxseed
- 1 cup or red grapes

Day 6:

- 1 tablespoon of ground flaxseed
- Meal replacement shake
- 1 cup of frozen blueberries

Day 7:

- 1 cup of yogurt

- 1 tablespoon of dried cranberries
- 6 hardboiled egg whites
- 1 tablespoon of ground flaxseed

Sample Morning Snack Recipe

Chocolate and Peanut Butter Parfait

This is another healthy bodybuilding meal plan best suited for those who have a sweet tooth. There are around eight ingredients that you will need, namely:

- 1 scoop of Gaspari ISO Fusion protein powder
- 1 tablespoon of cocoa powder
- 1 tablespoon of an instant coffee powder
- Fresh blueberries
- 1 cup of Greek yogurt that is non-fat
- 2 tablespoons of powdered peanut butter
- 1/3 cup of organic granola
- 1 tablespoon of dark chocolate chips.

Making a healthy chocolate peanut butter parfait with blueberries is simple.

1. Add the granola into a jar, bowl, or cup.
2. Add the yogurt and mix it with the granola, One by one, add the peanut butter powder, coffee, and cocoa into the jar, along with cups of non-fat Greek yogurt.
3. Finally, top it with dark chocolate chips, granola, and blueberries. You now have your protein-filled chocolate and peanut butter parfait with blueberries and chocolate chips. You may leave it in the refrigerator for a while before eating. It tastes good whether frozen or not.

Chapter 11 – What Not to Eat

Now that the mentioned meal plans have helped you decide on what kinds of meals you should prepare, the next important thing that you should know are the kinds of food that you must avoid. Remember that the unhealthiest foods are also among the most tempting. This chapter will share the kinds of food that will make you unhealthy and will hinder you from achieving the body and condition that you aspire for. They are as follows:

Soda. Although some of types say that they are a "diet soda" or have no fat, believe me when I say that these sodas are full of sugar. Soda is not soda without sugar. Sugar is not only a hindrance to bodybuilding, but an excessive amount can also cause serious health risks. Start avoiding this drink by making your own fruit juice. Glasses of water are also enough to keep you going.

Trans Fat. Foods with too much trans fat are unhealthy. These are the kinds of food that are too greasy, such as pizza. They may be very tempting to eat, but you must avoid them. They increase bad cholesterol while lowering good cholesterol. They bring serious risks and complications, and they could even trigger stroke.

Too Much Milk. Milk is healthy but not when taken in excessive amounts. Milk has lactose and sugar that are unhealthy for your body. Lactose makes it difficult for you to digest food. Do not wait until you have digestive issues when you can simply minimize your intake of milk.

Chocolate. It tastes really good but it is a big no-no for bodybuilders. It does not only contain too much sugar, it also has caffeine. It keeps you from sleeping at the right time, and it hinders you from recovering from your workout sessions. Lack of sleep caused by caffeine may lead to muscle tissue breakdown. As mentioned earlier, too much sugar is also bad for the health.

These are just some of the foods that you need to avoid. There are alternatives to these foods that are healthier and risk-free. Make sure that you do not include large amounts of these kinds of food in your meal plan so that you can successfully achieve your bodybuilding goals in no time.

Chapter 12 – Breakfast Recipes

Savory Whey Protein Crepes

Calories - 55, Fat - 1 g, Carbohydrates - 1 g, Protein - 10 g

Ingredients

- 1 cup egg whites
- ¼ cup unsweetened whey protein powder
- 2 heaped tablespoons coconut flour
- ¼ cup milk of your choice
- ½ teaspoon paprika
- ½ teaspoon garlic salt or to taste
- ½ teaspoon Italian seasoning
- Cooking spray or coconut oil or butter
- Filling of your choice

Method

1. Blend together all the ingredients in a blender until smooth.
2. Place a nonstick pan over medium heat. Spray with cooking spray. Add about ¼ cup of the batter on the center of the pan. Spread the batter around the pan with the back of a spoon to get a thin crepe.

3. When the bottom side is cooked to light brown, flip sides and cook the other side too.

4. Repeat steps 2 and 3 for the rest of the batter.

5. Place the filling in the center, fold over and serve.

Breakfast Burritos

Calories - 313, Fat - 10 g, Carbohydrates - 30 g, Protein -24.4 g

Ingredients

- 2 whole wheat tortilla (8 inch each)
- 2 whole eggs
- 6 egg whites
- 2 lettuce leaves
- ¼ cup fat free refried beans
- 2 tablespoons reduced fat cheddar cheese, shredded
- ½ cup salsa, divided

Method

1. Whisk together eggs and egg whites.
2. Place a nonstick pan over medium heat. Spray with cooking spray. Warm the tortillas on it one by one and place on individual plates.
3. To the same pan, pour the beaten eggs over it. Cook until the eggs are set. Stir a couple of times in between.
4. Meanwhile, place a lettuce leaf each over the tortillas. Spread half the beans over each of the lettuce leaf.
5. Divide the eggs amongst the 2 tortillas and place over the beans. Sprinkle cheddar cheese.
6. Finally, top each with 2 tablespoons of salsa. Roll and serve with the remaining salsa.

Blueberry Muffins

Calories - 206, Fat - 9 g, Carbohydrates - 25 g, Protein - 9 g

Ingredients

- 3 cups flour
- ½ cup stevia
- 4 teaspoons baking powder
- 2 teaspoons baking soda
- 1 teaspoon soda
- 1 teaspoon ground cinnamon
- 4 egg whites
- 6 ripe bananas, peeled, mashed
- 1 cup fresh blueberries
- 2/3 cup almond milk
- 2 cups applesauce, sugar free
- ½ cup vanilla caramel whey protein powder
- 2 cups walnuts, chopped

Method

1. Mix together in a large bowl, all the dry ingredients.
2. Mix together rest of the ingredients (wet ingredients) in another large bowl.

3. Add the dry ingredient mixture to the wet ingredients and mix well.
4. Add blueberries and walnuts. Fold gently.
5. Pour into greased muffin tins (fill it up to ¾).
6. Bake in a preheated oven at 350 degree F for about 20-25 minutes or until a toothpick when inserted in the center comes out clean.

Early Riser Breakfast

Calories -407g, Fat - 2 g, Carbohydrates - 46 g, Protein - 52 g

Ingredients

- 9 egg whites, whisked well
- 4 thick asparagus spears, sliced
- ½ cup cooked brown rice
- ½ cup cooked quinoa
- 1 medium red bell pepper, sliced
- ½ teaspoon garlic powder
- ½ teaspoon pepper powder
- Sea salt to taste
- ¾ pink grapefruit
- 1 ½ scoops whey protein
- Cooking spray with coconut oil or olive oil

Method

1. Spray an oven proof baking dish or cast iron skillet with cooking spray.
2. Add brown rice and oats to it. Add egg whites and spread it all over.
3. Lay the slices of bell pepper all over the egg whites. Lay the asparagus strips all over the egg whites.

4. Bake in a preheated oven at 405 degree F for around15 minutes or until the eggs are set.
5. Serve hot immediately.

Quinoa Pancakes

Calories - 182.4 g, Fat - 9 g, Carbohydrates - 22.3 g, Protein - 4 g

Ingredients

- 3 cups quinoa flour
- 1 ½ teaspoon baking powder
- ¾ teaspoon baking soda
- 3 teaspoons ground cinnamon
- 2 ½ to 3 cups non-dairy milk
- 3 tablespoons maple syrup
- 1 ½ teaspoons vanilla extract
- Egg substitute for 3 eggs
- Topping of your choice like berries, nuts, chocolate chips etc.
- Cooking spray

Method

1. Mix together all the dry ingredients in a large bowl.
2. Add vanilla, maple syrup and egg substitute. Mix well. Slowly pour in the milk. Mix well to get a smooth batter.
3. Add a little topping to the batter. Mix well and keep aside for a while.
4. Place a nonstick pan over medium heat. Spray with cooking spray. Add about 2 tablespoons of the batter on

the pan. If you have a large pan, you can make a few at a time in batches.

5. Cook until the bottom side is golden brown. Flip sides and cook the other side too. Remove and keep warm in an oven.
6. Repeat with the remaining batter.

Tofu Scramble

Calories - 159, Fat - 9.1 g, Carbohydrates - 11.9 g, Protein - 11 g

Ingredients

- 2 packages firm or extra firm tofu
- 2 large heads broccoli, chopped finely
- 4 cloves garlic, minced
- 1 avocado, peeled, pitted, chopped
- 2 injera, torn into pieces (optional)
- 1 teaspoons Berbere (Ethiopian spice blend) or to taste
- 1 teaspoon curry powder
- 1 teaspoon Hungarian paprika
- 1 teaspoon cumin
- ½ teaspoon dried thyme
- A large pinch cinnamon
- A large pinch ground cardamom
- A large pinch allspice
- A large pinch ground cloves
- 1 teaspoon salt, or to taste
- 1 tablespoon coconut oil

Method

1. Place a skillet over medium heat. Add coconut oil. When the oil is heated, add broccoli, and garlic and sauté for a couple for minutes.

2. Add tofu and sauté until brown. Stir constantly to prevent sticking.

3. Mix together in a bowl, berbere, a little water (2-3 tablespoons), curry powder, cardamom, cinnamon, cloves, thyme, paprika, thyme, cumin and allspice. Add it to the pan and mix well.

4. Add injera. Sauté for a couple of minutes until the mixture is almost dry.

5. Add avocado, mix well and serve.

Chocolate Cream Pancakes

Calories - 351, Fat - 5 g, Carbohydrates - 10 g, Protein - 2 g

Ingredients

For the pancakes

- ¼ cup buckwheat flour
- ¼ cup pea protein powder
- 2 tablespoons ground flax seeds
- 3 tablespoons apple cider vinegar
- ½ teaspoon baking powder
- Stevia to taste
- 1 cup cannellini beans
- 1 teaspoon coconut oil + more if required

For the chocolate cream

- 2 tablespoons flaxseed oil
- 2 tablespoons cocoa powder
- 2 tablespoons agave nectar

Method

1. Mix together in a bowl, buckwheat flour, pea protein, flax seeds, vinegar, baking powder, and stevia and about ½ a cup of water.

2. Add beans and mix well. Transfer the entire contents of the bowl to a food processor and process until the beans are mashed up.
3. Place a nonstick frying pan over medium heat. Add coconut oil. Add about ½ a cup of the pancake mixture on the pan. Spread it a bit. If your pan is large, then you can make 2-3 at a time.
4. When the bottom side is golden brown, flip the pancake and cook the other side too.
5. To make the chocolate cream: Mix together all the ingredients well.
6. Serve warm pancakes with the chocolate cream. Serve with fruits of your choice.

Breakfast Fajitas

Calories - 470, Fat - 27 g, Carbohydrates - 6 g, Protein - 12 g

Ingredients

- 12 egg whites, beaten
- 2 yolks, beaten
- 6 fat free whole wheat flour tortillas
- 1 cup fat free cheddar cheese
- 1 cup salsa
- Cooking spray

Method

1. Place a skillet over medium heat. Spray with cooking spray.
2. Mix together the whites and yolks. Pour the eggs in the skillet. When the eggs are slightly set, scramble it and cook until done. Remove from heat and add cheddar cheese.
3. Warm the tortillas. Place the egg mixture amongst the tortillas. Roll it up. Top with salsa and serve.

Chapter 13 – Lunch Recipes

Healthy Pita Pizza

Calories - 312, Fat - 34 g, Carbohydrates - 31 g, Protein - 24 g

Ingredients

- 2 large pitas
- ½ cup pizza sauce
- ½ cup part skim mozzarella, shredded
- 6 ounces (2 links) sweet Italian chicken sausage, remove the casing
- ½ cup sliced mushrooms
- ½ cup sliced bell pepper
- 2 tablespoons Parmesan, grated
- A large pinch crushed red pepper flakes

Method

1. Place a pan over medium heat. Add the sausages. Cook until brown. Break up the sausages while cooking.
2. Place the pita bread on a greased baking sheet. Bake in a preheated oven at 400 degree F for about 8-10 minutes.
3. Remove the baking sheet from the oven. Spread the pita bread with pizza sauce. Sprinkle mushrooms and bell peppers all over.

4. Bake at 500 degree F for 5-7 minutes. Finally sprinkle cheese.

5. Serve sprinkled with red pepper flakes.

Baked Potato Oatmeal

Calories - 329, Fat - 7 g, Carbohydrates - 45 g, Protein - 22 g

Ingredients

- 1 ½ cups rolled oats, cooked according to instructions on the package
- 1 ½ cups red potatoes, scrubbed, cubed
- 4 slices turkey bacon, uncured
- 2 tablespoons low fat cheddar cheese, shredded
- ¼ cup 2% Greek yogurt
- ½ teaspoon garlic salt
- ½ teaspoon black pepper powder
- Salt to taste
- 2 green onions, chopped

Method

1. Place the potatoes in a greased baking dish. Sprinkle salt, garlic salt, and pepper.
2. Bake in a preheated oven at 400 degree F for about 20 minutes until the potatoes are soft.
3. Meanwhile, place a skillet over medium heat. Add the bacon and cook until brown. Remove from pan and cool. When cooled, chop into small pieces.
4. Mix together the oats, cheddar cheese, potatoes, bacon and yogurt. Sprinkle salt and pepper.

5. Garnish with green onions.

Chicken & Broccoli Casserole

Calories - 466, Fat - 12 g, Carbohydrates - 35 g, Protein - 56 g

Ingredients

- 30 ounces chicken breast, cooked
- 3 cups 2% Greek yogurt
- 2 cups chicken broth + more if necessary
- 2 cups reduced-fat mozzarella, shredded
- 4 cups quinoa & brown rice mix, cooked
- 4 cups raw broccoli, chopped
- ½ cup red onion
- 1 cup crushed amaranth flakes,
- 1 cup wheat breadcrumbs, or panko crumbs
- 2 tablespoons Italian seasoning
- Sea salt to taste
- Pepper powder to taste

Method

1. Place a nonstick skillet over medium heat. Add chicken breasts and cook until done. When cool enough to handle, use a fork and make it into smaller pieces.
2. Mix together in a bowl the chicken, broccoli, brown rice and quinoa mix, red onions, Greek Yogurt, chicken broth, mozzarella and Italian seasoning.

3. Transfer into a casserole dish. Spread a layer of wheat bread crumbs all over the dish. Sprinkle amaranth flakes.
4. Bake in a preheated oven at 375 degree F for about 25-30 minutes or until done.

High Protein Mac & Cheese

Calories - 253, Fat - 8 g, Carbohydrates - 27 g, Protein - 20 g

Ingredients

- 8 slices turkey bacon, cured, nitrate free, sliced
- 9 ounces whole wheat macaroni or gluten-free quinoa macaroni, cooked according to the instructions on the package
- 3 ½ cups 2% Greek yogurt, divided
- 4 ounces goat cheese
- 1 cup reduced fat mozzarella
- 2 tablespoons garlic paste
- Fresh chives
- Sea salt to taste
- Black pepper to taste

Method

1. Place a nonstick skillet over medium high heat. Add bacon and cook for a couple of minutes.
2. Add garlic paste and cook until bacon is brown.
3. Lower the heat to medium. Add about 2 cups of yogurt, goat cheese, chives and mozzarella.
4. Cook until the sauce is thickened.

5. Remove from heat and macaroni. Add the remaining Greek yogurt. Mix well and serve.

Curry Shrimps on Rice

Calories -223, Fat - 1.2 g, Carbohydrates - 28 g, Protein - 23 g

Ingredients

- 3 cups cooked rice
- 1 teaspoon dried oregano
- Salt to taste
- 1 ½ pounds large shrimp, peeled, cooked
- 1 teaspoon curry powder
- ½ teaspoon cayenne pepper
- 1 large tomato, sliced

Method

1. Sprinkle salt and oregano over the rice.
2. Sprinkle curry powder and cayenne pepper over the shrimps.
3. Place the shrimps at the center on a serving platter. Place the rice all around the shrimps.
4. Serve with tomatoes.

Chicken Fried Rice

Calories -329, Fat - 11.96 g, Carbohydrates -41.82 g, Protein - 12.45 g

Ingredients

- 6 ounce chicken breasts, diced
- 1 cup brown rice, rinsed
- 4 egg whites
- 1 green bell pepper, chopped
- 1 red bell pepper, chopped
- 1 large onion, chopped
- 1 cup mushrooms, chopped
- 1 1/2 cups chicken broth
- 1 tablespoon soy sauce
- 1 tablespoon olive oil

Method

1. Place a skillet over medium heat. Add 1/2-tablespoon oil. When the oil is heated, add chicken pieces. Cook until tender. Remove from the skillet and transfer to a bowl. Keep aside.

2. To the same pan, add the remaining olive oil. Add the egg whites. Stir constantly until it is cooked. Remove from the pan and transfer it to the chicken bowl.

3. Add chicken broth and soy sauce to a saucepan and bring to a boil over medium heat.
4. Lower heat. Add bell peppers, onions, mushrooms, and rice. Mix well.
5. Cover and simmer until the rice is cooked.
6. Transfer the chicken and egg whites back to the skillet and fry for a few minutes until crisp.
7. Serve the chicken and egg whites over the rice.

Chapter 14 – Dinner Recipes

Grilled Fish Tacos

Calories - 468 g, Fat - 21 g, Carbohydrates - 37 g, Protein - 31 g

Ingredients

- 2 tablespoons olive oil
- 8 limes, halved, divided
- 10 cloves garlic, minced, divided
- 4 teaspoons ground cumin, divided
- 3 pounds swordfish or tuna
- 2 ripe avocadoes, peeled, pitted, diced
- ½ red onion, minced
- 4 jalapenos, seeded, minced
- 4 tablespoons fresh cilantro, chopped
- 16 flour tortillas (6 inch each)
- 16 lettuce leaves

Method

1. To marinate the fish: Mix together in a large bowl, olive oil, juice of 6 limes, 8 cloves garlic and 2 teaspoons cumin.

2. Add the fish and mix well. Keep aside for about 15-20 minutes. Turn the fish around a couple of times in between.
3. Meanwhile make the salsa as follows: Mix together in a small bowl, 2 cloves garlic, juice of 2 lime and 2 teaspoons cumin.
4. Add avocado, onions, jalapenos and cilantro. Mix well.
5. Place the fish on a preheated grill and the fish for around 5 minutes. Then turn the fish to cook the other side too. Cook for about 5 minutes or until the fish is opaque.
6. Remove and keep the fish on a cutting board. When it is cool enough to handle, slice into thin long pieces.
7. Warm the tortillas over the warm grill for a few seconds on both the sides.
8. To serve: Place a lettuce leaf over each tortilla. Place some fish over it. Spread some salsa over it. Fold the tortillas and serve.

Sesame and Salmon Burgers

Calories - 420, Fat - 19 g, Carbohydrates - 40 g, Protein - 24 g

Ingredients

- 2 cans salmon, skinless, boneless
- ½ cup dry oats
- 2 tablespoons lemon juice
- 2 teaspoons minced ginger
- 2 tablespoons light soy sauce
- ½ cup sesame seeds
- ½ cup fat-free mayonnaise
- 2 tablespoons olive oil
- 6 whole wheat buns
- 2 cups spinach leaves

Method

1. Mix together in a bowl, salmon, soy sauce, lemon juice, oats, ginger, and mayonnaise.
2. Shape into patties. Press some sesame seeds in the patties.
3. Place a pan over medium heat. Add heat about a tablespoon of oil in it. Place a few of the patties on it. Fry on both the sides until golden brown.
4. Serve the patties over whole-wheat bun and spinach leaves. Serve with mustard.

Tuna Wraps

Only wraps: Calories - 64, Fat - 1.5 g, Carbohydrates - 5 g, Protein - 8 g

Ingredients

For the wraps

- ½ cup unflavored whey protein powder
- 2 whole large eggs
- 2 large egg whites
- 4 tablespoons psyllium husk powder
- 4 tablespoons buckwheat flour
- ½ cup milk of your choice
- Sea salt to taste
- 1 tablespoon tarragon
- Cooking spray

For the filling

- 2 cans tuna
- 10 olives chopped
- Sea salt to taste
- 1 teaspoon tarragon
- 2 -3 tablespoons low fat mayonnaise

Method

1. Blend together all the ingredients of the wraps until smooth.
2. Place a nonstick pan over high heat. Spray with coconut oil.
3. Pour about ¼ cup of the batter on the center of the pan. Spread the mixture with the back of a spoon to form a thin wrap.
4. When the underside is cooked, flip sides and cook the other side too. Do not overcook.
5. Repeat steps 2-4 with the remaining batter.
6. To make the filling: Mix together all the ingredients of the filling.
7. To serve: Place some of the filling at the center of the wraps. Roll over and serve.

Piri Piri Chicken Livers

Calories - 329.5 g, Fat - 19 g, Carbohydrates - 4.7 g, Protein - 42.8 g

Ingredients

- 2 pounds chicken livers, washed, cubed
- 2 teaspoons paprika
- 2 cloves garlic
- 2 onions, sliced
- 5 tablespoons lemon juice
- 2 red bell peppers, sliced
- 4 handfuls baby spinach
- 1 teaspoon piri piri spice
- 1 teaspoon allspice
- 4 tablespoons olive oil
- 1 cup parsley, chopped
- Salt to taste
- 2 cups cooked rice

Method

1. Place a pan over medium heat. Add oil. When the oil is heated, add onions and garlic. Sauté until the onions are translucent.

2. Add red pepper. Sauté until the onions are brown.
3. Add chicken livers, piri piri spice, paprika and salt. Cook for 7-8 minutes.
4. Add spinach. Cook until the spinach wilts.
5. Place the rice over a serving platter. Pour the cooked chicken livers over it. Garnish with parsley and serve.

Chicken Enchiladas

Calories - 229.4, Fat - 8 g, Carbohydrates - 21.8 g, Protein - 17.4 g

Ingredients

- 2 pounds chicken breasts, cooked in water, shredded
- 8 green onions, sliced
- 1/4 cup fresh cilantro, chopped
- 2 jalapenos, seeded, minced
- 6 cans (10 ounce each) green enchilada sauce
- 16 corn tortillas
- 2 cups reduced fat cheddar cheese, shredded
- 4 cups lettuce, shredded
- 1 cup salsa
- 1 cup light sour cream
- 2 tomatoes, diced
- 2 cans (2 ounce each) ripe olives, sliced
- 1 tablespoon olive oil

Method

1. Place a large skillet over medium heat. Add olive oil. When oil is heated, add green onions, cilantro, and jalapeno. Stir-fry for a couple of minutes.

2. Add chicken and 2 cans of enchilada sauce. Heat thoroughly.
3. Pour the remaining cans of enchilada sauce in a microwavable bowl. Microwave on high for 2 minutes.
4. Dip a tortilla in the heated sauce. Place a little of the filling in it. Roll it up and place in a baking dish with its seam side down.
5. Repeat step 4 with the remaining tortillas.
6. Spread the remaining sauce over the tortillas.
7. Sprinkle cheddar cheese over the tortillas.
8. Bake in a preheated oven at 350 degree F until heated thoroughly and the cheese is melted.
9. To serve: Divide the lettuce amongst the tortillas and place in plates
10. Place the tortillas over the lettuce. Spread a spoonful of salsa over each of the tortillas. Top with tomatoes, olives, sour cream and serve.

Sweet Potato Lasagna

Calories - 381, Fat - 14.7 g, Carbohydrates - 39.6 g, Protein - 25.3 g

Ingredients

- 3 pounds lean ground turkey
- 1 1/2 pounds sweet potatoes, peeled, thinly sliced
- 2 egg whites
- 1 cup low fat cottage cheese
- 1 cup reduced fat mozzarella, shredded
- 4 wine tomatoes
- 2 cans (15 ounce each) tomato sauce, unsalted
- 2/3 cup mushrooms, sliced
- 2/3 cup red onions, chopped
- 2 tablespoons garlic paste
- 1 cup cilantro, chopped
- 2 tablespoons Italian seasoning
- Sea salt to taste
- Pepper powder to taste
- 1 tablespoon olive oil

Method

1. Mix together in a bowl, cottage cheese and egg whites. Keep aside.
2. Place a pan over medium heat. Add olive oil. When the oil is heated, add onions. Sauté for a couple of minutes.
3. Add garlic paste. Sauté for a while until the garlic is fragrant.
4. Add ground turkey, tomatoes, mushrooms, cilantro, tomato sauce, pepper, salt and Italian seasoning.
5. To assemble the lasagna: Lay the slices of sweet potato in a greased baking dish. Spread half the meat mixture.
6. Next spread half the cottage mixture over it.
7. Repeat steps 5 and 6 with the remaining mixtures.
8. Sprinkle mozzarella cheese all over. Cover the top of the dish with aluminum foil.
9. Bake in a preheated oven at 375 degree F for 45 minutes.
10. Serve immediately.

Chapter 15 – Vegetarian Recipe Options

Spicy Freekeh Chili

Calories - 215, Fat - 3 g, Carbohydrates - 41 g, Protein - 11 g

Ingredients

- 3 cups cooked Freekeh or quinoa, cooked according to the instructions on the package
- 1 ½ cans (15 ounce each can) tomato sauce, unsalted
- 3 vine tomatoes
- 3 cups low-sodium vegetable broth, divided
- 1 ½ cans (15 ounce each can) dark red kidney beans
- 1 ½ cans (15 ounce each) black beans
- 3 ½ cups frozen corn
- 2 cups red onion, chopped
- 4 garlic cloves, chopped
- 2 cups cilantro, chopped
- 2 tablespoons smoked paprika
- 1 ½ teaspoons coriander
- 1 ½ teaspoons chipotle chili pepper

- 1 ½ teaspoons ground cumin
- Cooking spray with coconut oil

Method

1. Place a large nonstick skillet over medium heat. Spray with cooking spray.
2. Add onions and garlic and sauté until the onions are brown.
3. Add tomato sauce, Freekeh, half the broth, bell pepper, tomatoes, paprika, coriander, chipotle chili pepper, and cumin powder. Mix well.
4. Add beans, corn, cilantro and the remaining broth.
5. Lower heat and simmer for about 15 minutes.
6. Garnish with a little cilantro and serve hot.

Tofu in Sauce

Calories - 329, Fat - 18 g, Carbohydrates - 27 g, Protein - 20 g

Ingredients

- ½ cup brown sugar
- ½ cup soy sauce
- 2 teaspoons chili flakes
- 4 teaspoons sesame oil
- 4 cloves garlic, minced
- 2 teaspoons fresh ginger, grated
- Salt to taste
- 124 ounce tofu, chopped
- 2 teaspoons olive oil

Method

1. Place a skillet over medium heat. Add olive oil. When the oil is hot, add tofu and cook until light brown.
2. Add rest of the ingredients to the skillet and mix well. Cook until thoroughly heated.
3. Serve over cooked brown rice.

Lentil Marinara Spaghetti Squash

Calories -140, Fat - 16 g, Carbohydrates - 20.3 g, Protein -8 g

Ingredients

- 2 whole spaghetti squash
- 2 cans diced Tomatoes
- 2 cups cooked lentils
- 2 tablespoons olive oil
- 2 cups broccoli, chopped
- 1 onion, chopped
- 1 red bell pepper, chopped
- 2 tablespoons garlic, chopped
- 2 tablespoons Italian seasoning
- Salt to taste
- Black pepper to taste

Method

1. Prick the squash with a fork all over.
2. Place the squash in a greased baking dish and bake for an hour at 400 degree F in a preheated oven. When done, remove from oven and keep aside to cool.

3. To make the lentil marinara sauce: Place a large skillet over medium heat. Add olive oil. When the oil is heated, add garlic and sauté for a couple of minutes.

4. Add lentils, tomatoes, broccoli, bell pepper, onions, salt, pepper, and Italian seasoning. Mix well and bring to a boil.

5. Lower heat and simmer for 15 – 20 minutes.

6. Meanwhile, remove the pulp of the spaghetti squash with a fork and place on a serving plate.

7. Pour the lentil marina sauce over the squash and serve.

Layered Portabella Mushrooms

Calories - 324, Fat - 14.5, Carbohydrates - 34 g, Protein - 18.25 g

Ingredients

- 4 large Portabella mushroom caps, cleaned, rinsed, pat dried
- 1 cup cooked quinoa
- 1 cup tempeh, crumbled
- 1 onion, diced
- 2 cups spinach
- 2 tomatoes, sliced
- ¼ almond cheese or fat free mozzarella, shredded
- 2 tablespoons olive oil
- 1 tablespoon paprika
- 1 tablespoon ground cumin
- 1 tablespoon garlic powder
- 1 tablespoon onion powder
- Sea salt to taste
- Pepper powder to taste

Method

1. Place a skillet over medium heat. Add olive oil. When the oil is heated, add onions. Sauté for a couple of minutes.
2. Add tempeh and sauté for 3-4 minutes. Add quinoa, salt, pepper, paprika, cumin, garlic powder and onion powder. Mix well.
3. Place portabella mushrooms over a lined baking sheet. Brush the mushrooms with olive oil.
4. Place spinach over each of the mushrooms. Layer the quinoa mixture over the spinach. Next place the tomatoes over the quinoa and finally top with shredded cheese.
5. Broil in a preheated oven for about 5 minutes.

Tofu Bento

Calories - 257, Fat - 8 g, Carbohydrates - 13 g, Protein - 18 g

Ingredients

- 2 packages extra firm tofu, pressed of excess moisture, pat dried, chopped
- 4 cups cooked brown rice
- ¼ cup low sodium soy sauce
- 2 teaspoons ginger, grated
- 2 teaspoons garlic powder
- 2 teaspoons onion powder
- 2 teaspoons chili paste
- 2 bunches broccolini, chopped
- 1 red bell pepper, sliced
- 1 green bell pepper, sliced
- 1 yellow bell pepper, sliced
- 1 orange bell pepper sliced
- ½ cup green onion, sliced (optional)
- Sriracha sauce to taste

Method

1. Place a large skillet over medium heat. Add olive oil. When the oil is heated, add broccolini and bell peppers. Sauté until slightly soft. Remove from heat.

2. Place another pan over medium heat. Add tofu and sauté until light brown.

3. To serve: Place some brown rice over individual serving plates. Place some tofu over the rice. Top with vegetables. Garnish with green onions.

Spinach with Pasta

Calories - 671, Fat - 21.4 g, Carbohydrates -93.6 g, Protein - 33 g

Ingredients

- 2 cups portabella mushroom caps, sliced
- 8 ounces vegetarian sausages, chopped
- 1 cup onions, chopped
- 1/2 cup red wine
- 2 tablespoons olive oil
- 2 cloves garlic, minced
- Salt to taste
- Black pepper powder to taste
- 1 teaspoon oregano
- 2 ounce whole wheat penne pasta, cook according to the instructions on the package
- 4 cups spinach leaves
- 2 tablespoons balsamic vinegar

Method

1. Place a large skillet over medium heat. Add olive oil. When the oil is heated, add onions, garlic. Sauté for a couple of minutes. Add mushrooms and sauté for a while

until the vegetables are slightly brown.

2. Add red wine. Mix well.
3. Add sausages, salt, pepper and oregano. Add pasta and toss.
4. To serve: Place the spinach over a serving platter. Place the pasta along with the sausages over the spinach. Sprinkle balsamic vinegar and serve.

Chapter 16 – Smoothie Recipes

Breakfast Shake

Calories - 599, Fat - 12 g, Carbohydrates - 46 g, Protein - 57 g

Ingredients

- 3 cups skim milk
- ¾ cup frozen strawberries
- 3 scoops whey protein
- 1 ½ cups oatmeal
- 2 tablespoons flax seeds

Method

1. Blend together all the ingredients until smooth.
2. Serve in tall glasses with crushed ice.

Banana and Almond Cream Shake

Calories - 320, Fat - 8 g, Carbohydrates - 32 g, Protein - 32 g

Ingredients

- 1 scoop pea protein
- 1 scoop rice protein
- 2 bananas, peeled, chopped
- 1 cup skim milk
- 20 almonds

Method

1. Blend together all the ingredients until smooth.
2. Serve in tall glasses with crushed ice.

Green Monster

Calories - 497, Fat - 17 g, Carbohydrates - 62 g, Protein - 28 g

Ingredients

- 4 bunches kale, stems removed, chopped
- 4 stalks celery, chopped
- 1 cup spinach, roughly chopped
- 5-6 slices pineapple, chopped
- 1 ½ tablespoons coconut oil
- 1 ½ scoops Monster milk vanilla crème
- 1 cup water

Method

1. Blend together all the ingredients until smooth.
2. Serve in tall glasses with crushed ice.

Pre-Workout Drink

Calories - 195, Fat - 0.7 g, Carbohydrates - 53.6 g, Protein - 4.1 g

Ingredients

- 6 stalks celery, chopped
- 4 medium apples, cored, peeled, chopped
- 1 cup water

Method

1. Blend together all the ingredients until smooth.
2. Serve in tall glasses with crushed ice.

Fruit Smoothie

Calories - 403, Fat - 4.9g, Carbohydrates - 77.5g, Protein - 16.5 g

Ingredients

- 2 large bananas, peeled, chopped
- 5 ounces sunflower seeds, soaked
- 1 cup strawberries, chopped
- 1 cup raspberries
- 1 cup blackberries
- 1 cup blueberries
- 2 cups water

Method

1. Blend together all the ingredients until smooth.
2. Serve in tall glasses with crushed ice.

Pina Colada

Calories -254, Fat - 11.1 g, Carbohydrates - 32.4 g, Protein - 8g

Ingredients

- 1 cup pineapple, chopped
- 1 frozen banana, chopped
- 2 scoops vanilla protein powder
- 1 cup coconut milk, unsweetened
- 1 cup water

Method

1. Blend together all the ingredients until smooth.
2. Serve in tall glasses with crushed ice.

Wild Berry Shake

Calories - 94.8, Fat - 0.5 g, Carbohydrates - 17.4 g, Protein - 6 g

Ingredients

- 4 scoops whey powder
- 15 strawberries
- 20 blueberries
- 20 raspberries
- 10 blueberries
- 4 cups nonfat milk

Method

1. Blend together all the ingredients until smooth.
2. Serve in tall glasses with crushed ice.

Chapter 17 – Soup Recipes

Spinach and Tofu Soup

Calories - 57.3, Fat - 2.5 g, Carbohydrates - 4.8 g, Protein - 6 g

Ingredients

- 6 inch block fresh tofu, chopped into 1 centimeter cubes
- 4 bunches spinach, rinsed, chopped into small pieces
- 6 cups vegetable stock
- 2 tablespoons light soy sauce
- Salt to taste
- Freshly ground black pepper to taste

Method

1. Place a large saucepan over medium heat. Pour the stock into it and bring it to a boil.
2. Add tofu, salt, pepper and soy sauce. Mix well and bring to a boil.
3. Add spinach and simmer for a couple of minutes until the spinach is wilted.
4. Taste and adjust the seasonings.
5. Ladle into individual soup bowls and serve immediately.

Muscle Building Chili

Calories - 420, Fat - 6.8 g, Carbohydrates - 50 g, Protein - 40.5 g

Ingredients

- 1 pound chicken breasts, chopped into bite sized pieces
- 1 tablespoon olive oil
- 1 green bell pepper, chopped
- 1 red bell pepper, chopped
- 1/2 cup mushrooms, sliced
- 1 medium onion, finely chopped
- 1/2 cup frozen corn kernels
- 1 can (15 ounce) light kidney beans
- 1 can (15 ounce) dark red kidney beans
- 1/2 a 15 ounce can pinto beans
- 1 cup barley (optional)
- 1 can (15 ounce) tomatoes
- 1/2 a 15 ounce can tomato sauce
- 2 cups water
- 1 teaspoon chili powder or to taste
- 1/2 teaspoon oregano
- 1 clove garlic, minced
- 1/2 teaspoon ground cumin
- 1/2 cup Worcestershire sauce
- Salt to taste

- 2-3 tablespoons low fat cheddar cheese

Method

1. Place a large saucepan over medium heat. Add olive oil. When the oil is heated, add garlic and sauté for a few seconds until fragrant.
2. Add onions, pepper and mushrooms. Sauté for a few minutes until onions are translucent.
3. Add chicken, all the types of beans, corn, tomatoes, tomatoes, and water. Mix well. Bring to a boil.
4. Add barley, cumin, chili powder, oregano, salt and Worcestershire sauce.
5. Reduce heat and simmer for about 20 minutes.
6. Garnish with cheddar cheese and serve hot.

Chicken Vegetable Soup

Calories - 84, Fat - 9 g, Carbohydrates - 7.7 g, Protein - 8.2 g

Ingredients

- 1 tablespoon olive oil
- 2 chicken breasts, chopped into small pieces
- 2 cloves garlic, minced
- 1 medium onion, chopped
- 1 stick celery, chopped
- 1 1/2 cups cabbage
- 2 carrots, peeled, chopped
- 1 small zucchini, chopped
- 3/4 cup baby corn
- 3/4 teaspoon dried oregano
- 3/4 teaspoon dried basil
- 3/4 teaspoon dried thyme
- 4 cups low sodium chicken broth
- 1 1/2 cups spinach, chopped
- 2 green onions, chopped
- Salt to taste
- Pepper powder to taste

Method

1. Place a large saucepan over medium heat. Add olive oil. When oil is heated, add onions and garlic. Sauté for a couple of minutes.
2. Add celery and carrots and sauté for a few minutes until it is tender.
3. Add zucchini, cabbage, baby corn and sauté for 2-3 minutes.
4. Add chicken, chicken broth, the dried herbs, salt and pepper. Bring to a boil.
5. Lower heat. Cover and simmer until the chicken is cooked.
6. Add green onion and spinach and cook for a couple of minutes until the spinach is wilted.

Oriental Noodle Soup

Calories - 83, Fat - 1.2 g, Carbohydrates - 5 g, Protein - 6.8 g

Ingredients

- 2 teaspoons vegetable oil
- 1 medium onion, chopped
- 2 cloves garlic, minced
- 1/2 tablespoon fresh ginger, minced
- 4 cups beef broth
- 2 carrots, peeled, chopped
- 1/2 cup broccoli florets
- 1/4 cup snow peas
- 1/2 cup celery, chopped
- 5 ounce shrimps, peeled, deveined
- 3 ounces rice vermicelli
- 1/2 tablespoon low sodium soy sauce
- 1/2 cup bean sprouts
- Pepper powder to taste

Method

1. Place a large saucepan over medium heat. Add olive oil. When the oil is heated, add onions, ginger and garlic.
2. Sauté for a couple of minutes until the onions are translucent.
3. Add beef broth, carrots, celery, carrots, snow peas, and broccoli. Mix well and bring it to a boil.

4. Lower the heat, cover and simmer until the vegetables are cooked.
5. Add rice vermicelli and cook until it is slightly soft.
6. Add shrimps. Cover again and simmer for 6-7 minutes.
7. Lastly, add the soy sauce, pepper powder. Mix well.
8. Ladle into individual bowls.
9. Top with bean sprouts and serve immediately.

Vegan Split Pea Soup

Calories - 204, Fat - 1 g, Carbohydrates - 37 g, Protein - 14 g

Ingredients

- 1 1/2 cups green split peas, rinsed, soaked in water overnight
- 1 medium white onion, chopped
- 1 large carrot, sliced
- 3 stalks celery, sliced
- 1 1/2 teaspoons ground cumin
- Sea Kelp delight seasoning to taste
- 4 tablespoons liquid aminos or to taste
- 14-15 cups water

Method

1. Place all the ingredients in a large pot. Place the pot over medium heat.
2. Cook until the split peas are tender. (You can also place all the ingredients in a crock-pot and set it on low for about 10-12 hours) Add more water if required.
3. Mix well. Ladle into bowls and serve hot.

Hearty Winter Vegetable Soup

Calories - 130, Fat - 0.6 g, Carbohydrates - 25.3 g, Protein - 7.3 g

Ingredients

- 1 cup red lentils, rinsed, soaked overnight
- 1/2 cup lima beans, rinsed, soaked overnight
- 1 onion, diced
- 8 cherry tomatoes, whole
- 1 medium carrot, peeled, sliced
- 2 stalks celery, sliced
- 1 small Serrano chili pepper, chopped
- 2 cloves garlic, minced
- 1/4 teaspoon paprika or to taste
- Sea salt to taste
- Pepper powder to taste
- 1/2 teaspoon curry powder or to taste
- 3 tablespoons liquid aminos or to taste
- 2 tablespoons parsley, chopped
- 4 cups water

Method

1. Place all the ingredients in a large pot. Place the pot over medium heat.

2. Cook until the split peas are tender. (You can also place all the ingredients in a crock-pot and set it on low for about 10-12 hours) Add more water if required.
3. Mix well. Ladle into bowls and serve hot.

Chapter 18 – Salad Recipes

Quinoa Salad

Calories - 141, Fat - 6 g, Carbohydrates - 16 g, Protein - 7 g

Ingredients

- 2 cups dry quinoa, cook according to the instructions on the package
- 2 cups shelled, frozen edamame
- 1 red bell pepper, sliced
- 1 yellow bell pepper, sliced
- 1/2 cup cilantro, chopped
- Juice of 2 limes
- 2 tablespoons olive oil
- 1 teaspoon garlic powder
- 1 teaspoon onion powder
- 1 teaspoon ground cumin
- 1 teaspoon paprika
- Salt to taste
- Pepper to taste
- 1 cup cooked black beans
- 1 red onion, chopped
- 2 tomatoes, chopped
- 1 cucumber, chopped

- 1/2 cup hummus (optional)

Method

1. Place a saucepan over medium heat. Add edamame and some water. Cook until the edamame is tender.
2. Fluff the cooked quinoa with a fork.
3. Add all the ingredients including quinoa and edamame to a large bowl. Mix well.
4. Keep aside for a while and then serve.

Tuna Salad with Fresh Dill

Calories - 158, Fat - 1 g, Carbohydrates - 7 g, Protein - 21 g

Ingredients

- 2 cans (7ounce each) of water-packed low-sodium tuna, rinsed and drained
- 1/2 cup celery, chopped
- 1/4 cup fresh dill, chopped
- 1/4 cup fresh parsley, chopped
- 1/2 cup nonfat yogurt
- 1 teaspoon low sodium Dijon mustard
- Pepper powder to taste
- A few lettuce leaves to serve

Method

1. Mix together all the ingredients in a bowl.
2. Place the lettuce leaves on a serving platter. Place the salad over the lettuce.
3. Serve with pita bread or baked potatoes.

Beet & Cucumber Salad

Calories - 96, Fat - 6 g, Carbohydrates - 12 g, Protein - 16 g

Ingredients

- 4 medium beets, peeled, chopped, steamed
- 2 medium cucumbers, chopped
- 1 cup sauerkraut
- 4 tablespoons rice wine vinegar
- 8 leaves Savoy cabbage (use it either raw or steamed)
- 2 teaspoons dried dill
- 1 cup almonds, soaked in water for 7-8 hours
- Sea salt to taste
- A large pinch of sugar

Method

1. Rinse the steamed beets with cold water. Drain and keep aside.
2. Place cucumber and sauerkraut in a bowl. Add dill and rice wine vinegar.
3. Add sugar and salt. Mix well and refrigerate until use.
4. To serve: Place the salad in the cabbage leaves. Place almonds over the salad and serve.

Apple & Nut Salad

Calories – 89, Fat - 6 g, Carbohydrates - 7 g, Protein - 11 g

Ingredients

- 2 heads red leaf lettuce
- 2 cups sunflower sprouts
- 2 apples, cored, diced
- 1 cup walnuts, chopped
- 2 cups grapes

Method

1. Place the lettuce leaves over a serving platter. Spread the sprouts over the lettuce.
2. Layer the apples, walnuts and grapes.
3. Serve immediately.

Power packed Salad

Calories - 167, Fat - 9 g, Carbohydrates - 9 g, Protein - 5 g

Ingredients

- 2 cups lettuce, torn into small pieces
- 1 cup spinach, torn into small pieces
- 1 small cucumber, peeled, sliced
- 1 tomato, sliced
- 1 1/2 cups sprouts
- 2/3 cup carrots, shredded
- 2/3 cup mushrooms, sliced
- 1/2 avocado, peeled, pitted, cubed
- 2 tablespoons raw sunflower seeds
- 2 tablespoons olive oil
- 2 tablespoons lemon juice
- 1/2 teaspoon dried thyme
- 1/2 teaspoon dried parsley
- 1/2 teaspoon dried basil

Method

1. Pour olive oil and lemon juice to a small jar that has a lid.
2. Add thyme, parsley and basil. Close the lid and shake until the mixture is well blended.

3. Add lettuce, cucumber, spinach, avocado, tomato, carrots, sprouts, mushrooms, and sunflower seeds to a bowl. Toss well.
4. Pour the dressing over the salad and serve.

Arugula Chicken Salad

Calories - 469, Fat - 12 g, Carbohydrates - 14 g, Protein - 65 g

Ingredients

- 2 tablespoons olive oil
- 20 baby carrots, chopped
- 1 cup red cabbage, chopped
- 2 cups arugula
- 16 ounce chicken, boneless, cubed
- Dressing of your choice (to taste)

Method

1. Place a pan over medium heat. Add olive oil. When the oil is heated, add the chicken cubes. Cook until the chicken is tender.
2. To a large salad bowl, add carrots, cabbage and arugula. Mix well.
3. Sprinkle the sunflower seeds. Top with chicken. Pour dressing on top and serve.

Mandarin and Kale Salad

Calories - 104, Fat - 4 g, Carbohydrates - 13 g, Protein - 4 g

Ingredients

- 8 cups kale, stems removed, cut into bite sized pieces
- 1/4 cups almonds, slivered
- 4 mandarin oranges, separated into segments
- 1/4 cup dried cranberries
- 1/4 cup olive oil
- 2 tablespoons vinegar
- 2 tablespoons honey

Method

1. Whisk together olive oil, vinegar and honey to make the dressing.
2. Add rest of the ingredients to a large bowl. Toss well.
3. Pour the dressing and serve immediately.

Chapter 19 – Snack Recipes

Peanut Butter Protein Bars

For 1 bar - Calories - 170, Fat - 8 g, Carbohydrates - 13.5 g, Protein - 6 g

Ingredients

- 1 cup skim milk
- 2 cups low fat peanut butter
- 2 tablespoons honey
- 3 cups chocolate cookie whey HD protein powder
- 4 cups dry, uncooked oatmeal (not the instant one)
- 2 tablespoons ground cinnamon
- ½ cup white yogurt chips

Method

1. Place a saucepan over low heat. Add peanut butter, honey and milk.
2. When the contents are warm, add protein powder and cinnamon and whisk well until well combined.
3. Add oats and stir. Add more milk if the mixture is very thick.
4. Transfer the contents to a greased pan. Press well.
5. Sprinkle the chips over it and press again so that the chips are stuck in the mixture.
6. When cooled, cut into bars and serve. Unused bars can be wrapped in cling wrap and refrigerated.

Grilled Pineapple

Calories - 67.1, Fat - 0.4 g, Carbohydrates - 17.1 g, Protein - 0.3 g

Ingredients

- 2 cans (8 ounce each) unsweetened pineapple slices (you can use fresh pineapple slices too)
- 2 large jalapenos, seeded, minced
- Juice of 2 lime
- ¼ teaspoon cayenne pepper
- A large pinch salt

Method

1. Preheat a grill and grill the pineapple pieces on both the sides until brown.
2. Once cool enough to handle, chop the pineapple slices into bite-sized pieces. Transfer into a bowl.
3. Add rest of the ingredients. Mix well. Cover and refrigerate for about an hour before serving. Stir in between a couple of times.

Fish Sticks

Calories - 133, Fat - 3 g, Carbohydrates - 9 g, Protein - 17 g

Ingredients

For the fish sticks

- 3 pounds halibut or cod, chopped into long pieces
- 1 cup panko breadcrumbs
- 4 tablespoons coconut flour
- 1 cup amaranth flakes, unsweetened
- ½ cup low fat parmesan, shredded
- 2 tablespoons Italian seasoning
- 2 teaspoons cayenne pepper
- 2 eggs, beaten
- 2 egg whites, beaten

For the sauce

- 1 cup low fat Greek yogurt
- ½ cup red onion, minced
- 1 teaspoon coriander
- Juice of a lemon
- Salt to taste
- Pepper powder to taste

Method

1. Mix together in a bowl, panko, amaranth flakes, coconut flour, Parmesan, Italian seasoning and cayenne pepper.
2. First dip the fish sticks in eggs; next roll the sticks in breadcrumbs and place on a greased baking sheet.
3. Bake in a preheated oven for 15 minutes.
4. To make the sauté. Mix together all the ingredients.
5. Serve the fish sticks with the sauce.

Shrimp Sliders

1 slider - Calories - 135, Fat - 2 g, Carbohydrates - 13 g, Protein - 14 g

Ingredients

- 12 ounce raw shrimps, deveined, peeled, remove tails
- A few multigrain slider buns
- 1 cup bell pepper, diced
- 2 roma tomatoes, sliced
- A few lettuce leaves
- 1 tablespoon coconut oil
- 1 teaspoon onion powder
- 1 teaspoon garlic powder
- Pepper powder to taste
- Salt to taste
- ½ teaspoon cumin powder

Method

1. Pat dry the shrimps with a paper towel and place in a food processor. Pulse until a paste is formed.
2. Transfer into a bowl. Add onion powder, garlic powder, cumin powder, and salt. Mix well and form into small patties (the size of the slider).
3. Place a nonstick pan over medium heat. Add a little coconut oil. Add a few of the patties. Fry on both the sides until pink.
4. Repeat step 3 with the remaining patties.

5. Place a small lettuce leaf over the slider. Place a slice of tomato over the lettuce and serve.

Cottage Cheese and Watermelon

Calories - 130.7, Fat - 1.9 g, Carbohydrates - 14.2 g, Protein - 15 g

Ingredients

- 3 cups low fat cottage cheese
- 2 cups water melon, cubed
- 2 tablespoons honey or to taste

Method

1. Mix together all the ingredients in a bowl.
2. Chill in the refrigerator.

Red Pear and Prosciutto Skewers

Calories - 118, Fat - 6 g, Carbohydrates - 12 g, Protein - 8 g

Ingredients

- 4 red pears, cut into triangular wedges
- 2 packages prosciutto
- 2-3 tablespoons balsamic vinegar

Method

1. Roll up the slices of prosciutto. Chop them into 2 halves each.
2. Thread the prosciuttos and pears alternately on to skewers.
3. Place on a serving platter. Sprinkle balsamic vinegar over it and serve.

Oatmeal Cookies

Calories - 673, Fat - 11 g, Carbohydrates - 121 g, Protein - 29 g

Ingredients

- 4 overripe bananas, peeled, mashed
- 2 cups oatmeal
- 1/4 teaspoon sea salt
- 2 teaspoons ground cinnamon
- 1/4 teaspoon baking powder
- 2 scoops Muscle Milk Vanilla Crème
- 1 tablespoon finely chopped almonds
- Cooking spray

Method

1. Add mashed bananas to bowl and beat well until creamy. Add oats, protein powder cinnamon, salt, baking powder and almonds.
2. Grease a baking sheet with cooking spray. Pour a spoonful of the batter (as much as the size of the cookie you want) all over the cookie sheet leaving a gap of about 1/2 inch between 2 cookies.
3. Bake in a preheated oven at 350 degree F for about 15 minutes.

Chapter 20 –Dessert Recipes

Chocó-berry Cheese cake

Calories - 216, Fat - 2 g, Carbohydrates - 33 g, Protein - 17 g

Ingredients

For the crust

- 1 ½ cups porridge oats
- 6 tablespoons almond milk
- ½ teaspoon cocoa powder
- A large pinch salt

For the cream

- 4 cups cannellini beans
- ½ cup almond milk
- 4 teaspoons stevia or any sweetener of your choice
- 2 scoops pea protein powder
- 1 teaspoon vanilla extract

For the chocolate layer

- 1 tablespoon cocoa powder
- 2 teaspoons stevia
- 2 tablespoons almond milk

For the berry layer

- 1 cup berries
- 2 teaspoons stevia
- 1 scoop pea protein powder

Method

1. To make the crust: Mix together all the ingredients of the crust. Transfer into a cake tin. Press well.
2. To make the cream: Add the cannellini beans, almond milk, stevia, pea protein powder and vanilla to a food processor. Pulse until well combined. Remove from the food processor and take out about a cup of the mixture and keep in a bowl. To this add the chocolate layer ingredients.
3. Spread this chocolate layer over the prepared crust.
4. To the remaining beans mixture, add berries and sweetener to it. Blend until smooth.
5. Spread over the chocolate layer.
6. Garnish with berries and sprinkle the coconut flakes.
7. Refrigerate until well chilled. Chop into slices and serve.

Oatmeal Carrot Cake

Calories - 292, Fat - 14 g, Carbohydrates - 37 g, Protein - 7 g

Ingredients

- 1 1/2 cups rolled oats, cooked according to instructions on the package
- 1/2 cup grated carrots + more for garnishing
- 1/4 cup almond milk
- 2 tablespoons raisins
- 2 packets stevia
- 1 teaspoon ground cinnamon
- 1/2 teaspoon allspice
- 2 -3 tablespoons coconut, shredded, toasted, for garnishing

Method

1. Cool the cooked oats and add to a serving bowl. Add rest of the ingredients and mix until well combined.
2. Garnish with shredded coconut and carrots and serve.

Maple Glazed Protein Doughnuts

Calories - 100, Fat - 3 g, Carbohydrates - 9 g, Protein - 11 g

Ingredients

For the doughnuts

- 2/3 cup oat flour
- 2 scoops vanilla flavored whey protein
- 1/2 cup baking stevia or 1/2 cup sugar free maple syrup
- 2 tablespoons coconut flour
- 1/4 cup ground flaxseed
- 1 teaspoon baking powder
- 1/2 cup + 2 tablespoons almond milk, unsweetened
- 1/2 cup egg whites
- 1/2 cup apple sauce, unsweetened
- 1/2 teaspoon butter extract (optional)
- 1/2 teaspoon maple extract

For frosting

- 1/2 cup sugar free maple syrup
- 2 scoops vanilla whey powder
- 1/2 teaspoon unflavored gelatin (optional)
- Sprinkles (optional) for garnishing

Method

1. To make the doughnuts: Mix together all the dry ingredients in a large bowl.
2. Add rest of the liquid ingredients. (If you are using maple syrup, then use only 1/2 cup of almond milk).
3. Mix thoroughly. Pour the batter into greased doughnut pans.
4. Bake in a preheated oven at 350 degree F for about 10 minutes. Remove from oven and cool slightly.
5. Invert on to a plate and keep aside to cool.
6. To make the frosting: Mix together all the ingredients of the frosting and refrigerate until thick.
7. Garnish with sprinkles and serve

Eggnog Ice cream

Calories - 179, Fat - 4.4 g, Carbohydrates - 7.8 g, Protein - 27.9 g

Ingredients

- 2 cups unsweetened vanilla almond milk
- 1/4 cup non-fat Greek yogurt
- 2 teaspoons ground nutmeg
- 4 tablespoons sugar-free Eggnog syrup
- 2 scoops vanilla protein

Method

1. Blend together all the ingredients.
2. Transfer into a freezable bowl, cover with cling film and freeze until done. Alternately place the ingredients in an ice cream machine and churn for 15-20 minutes.

Peach Chiffon

Calories - 176.7, Fat - 7.8 g, Carbohydrates - 28.6 g, Protein - 4.4 g

Ingredients

- 2 small packages peach Jell-O
- 3 cups boiling hot water
- 2 cups pecans
- 1/4 cup light butter
- 2/3 cup splenda
- 12 ounces ultra-low fat-free cream cheese
- 1 teaspoon vanilla extract
- 4 ripe peaches, pitted, sliced

Method

1. Add pecans to the food processor and pulse until coarse. Transfer into a bowl.
2. Add butter and splenda. Mix well.
3. Transfer into a large greased square pan. Spread the mixture all over the pan and press well.
4. Bake in a preheated oven at 300 degree F for about 7-8 minutes.
5. Meanwhile make the Jell- O according to the instructions on the package.
6. When the Jell - O is slightly beginning to set, transfer it to a blender or food processor.
7. Add cream cheese and vanilla and blend until smooth.

8. Pour over the baked crust.
9. Refrigerate until set.
10. Serve garnished with peach slices.

Chocolate Peanut Butter Fudge

Calories - 319, Fat – 11.8 g, Carbohydrates - 51 g, Protein – 11 g

Ingredients

- 16 ounces unsweetened baking chocolate squares
- 2 cups natural peanut butter
- 1/2 cup splenda or to taste
- 2 cups chocolate protein powder
- 1 cup peanuts, roasted, chopped

Method

1. Place the chocolate squares in a saucepan. Place the saucepan over low heat.
2. Stir constantly. When the chocolate is completely melted, add peanut butter and splenda. Mix well until well combined. Remove from heat.
3. Add protein powder, salt and 1/2 the peanuts. Transfer into a square pan.
4. Garnish with the remaining peanuts.
5. Refrigerate until use.

Protein Truffles

Calories - 63, Fat - 2.4 g, Carbohydrates - 3.85 g, Protein - 7 g

Ingredients

- 2 scoops whey protein
- 1/4 cup coconut flour
- 2 tablespoons cocoa powder
- 6 tablespoons unsweetened almond milk
- 1/4 cup shredded coconut, unsweetened

Method

1. Mix together in a bowl, whey protein coconut flour, cocoa powder and milk.
2. Shape into small balls.
3. Roll the balls in the shredded coconut and serve.

Conclusion

Thank you again for downloading this book!

I hope this book was able to help you plan your meals and bring you a few steps closer to achieving your bodybuilding goals.

The next step is to combine these nutrition programs and meal plans with your weightlifting exercises and other activities that are necessary for bodybuilding.

Finally, if you enjoyed this book, then I'd like to ask you for a favor, would you be kind enough to leave a review for this book on Amazon? It'd be greatly appreciated!

Thank you and good luck!

Made in the USA
San Bernardino, CA
30 November 2015